Copyright 2023

All right reserved. No part of this book should be resproduce without express permission of the author.

Reproduction of all or any part of this book is punishable under relevant law.

Table of Contents

Tinnitus is when you experience ringing or other noises in one or both of your ears. The noise you hear when you have tinnitus isn't caused by an external sound, and other people usually can't hear it. Tinnitus is a common problem. It affects about 15% to 20% of people, and is especially common in older adults.

Tinnitus is usually caused by an underlying condition, such as age-related hearing loss, an ear injury or a problem with the circulatory system. For many people, tinnitus improves with treatment of the underlying cause or with other treatments that reduce or mask the noise, making tinnitus less noticeable.

BREAKFAST

1. Keto Cheesecake – New York Baked Cheesecake

Prep Time: 20 Minutes

Cook Time: 50 Minutes

Servings: 12

Ingredient

Base

- 2 Cups Almond Flour 200g / 7 oz
- 1/2 Cup Coconut Flour 40g / 1.2 oz
- 6 oz unsalted butter must be cold (180g)
- 1 tsp baking powder
- 1/2 tsp Salt
- 1/2 tsp xanthan gum (optional)
- 2 Tbsp. Erythritol (So Nourished) granular

Filling:

- ◻2 Cups Cream Cheese full fat (500g / 1 lb)
- ◻3/4 Cup Sour Cream full fat

- ◻2/3 Cup Erythritol (So Nourished) granular

- ◻3 large Eggs

- ◻1 tsp Vanilla Extract

- ◻1 tsp Lemon Zest

Instructions

Base:

1. In a large glass bowl, mix the almond flour, coconut flour, xanthan gum, baking powder, erythritol and salt together until each of the ingredients are well combined.

2. This process has to be done quickly, otherwise, it will not work! – Cut the cold butter up into small chunks, and add it to the dry ingredients. Press the butter into the dry ingredients by using two forks. This can also be done in a food processor by pulsing the chunks of butter and dry ingredients for 20 – 30 seconds on high

3. In a 22cm (8.5") spring form cake tin, line the bottom insert with baking paper, grease the inside with butter and press the base mixture into the bottom of the tin. I usually press it halfway up the sides as well.

4. Place the tin in the fridge to allow the base to set. Preheat your oven to 140 degrees C (280 F) if fan forced, otherwise 160 degrees (320 F).

Filling:

1. In a mixing bowl, add the cream cheese, sour cream, vanilla extract, lemon zest and erythritol. Mix until well combined.

2. As the mixture begins to thicken slightly, add the first egg and continue to mix. Add in the rest of the eggs one at a time, and continue to mix.

3. Take the base out of the fridge, poke holes in the bottom of the base with a fork, and bake in the oven for 15 minutes until slightly golden. Remove and let cool slightly. Wrap the bottom of the tin in aluminum foil.

4. Using a sieve, pour the cream cheese filling through into the base (this helps remove any large clumps that might spoil the cheesecake). Put the cheesecake into the oven and bake in a large baking sheet filled with water (otherwise known as a water bath). Alternatively, you can place 2 ramekins filled with water right next to the cheesecake. Bake for 50 minutes.

5. Check the cheesecake by pushing a spike into the middle. If it comes out clean then the cake is ready.

6. Turn the oven off, and leave the oven slight open for another 30 mins to cool the cheesecake slowly. (This stops the top from cracking) Remove from the oven and let it come to room temperature before placing in the fridge for 4 hours to set. Keeps up to 5 days in an airtight container in the fridge.

Prep Time: 15 Minutes

Cook Time: 20 Minutes

Servings: 7

Ingredient

- 3/4 cup Peanut butter sugar free
- 2/3 cup Powdered Erythritol
- 1 Large Egg
- 1/2 tsp Vanilla Extract
- 1/2 tsp Salt
- 1/4 Cup Butter

Instructions

1. Preheat oven to 360F (180C). Make sure butter is soft, and mix all of the ingredients in a large bowl until well combined.
2. Roll them into 7 balls and squash flat with a fork
3. Bake for 15 – 20 mins until they start to turn slightly brown. Cool on a baking tray for 20 mins and enjoy!

Prep Time: 10 Minutes

Cook Time: 45 Minutes

Servings: 10

Ingredient

- Coconut Cake
- 1/2 Cup Coconut Flour 40g / 1.2 oz
- 5 large Eggs
- 1/4 Cup Erythritol (So Nourished) 30g / 1 oz
- 1/2 Cup Butter Melted 125g / 4 oz
- 1/2 Lemon Juiced
- 1/2 tsp Lemon Zest
- 1/2 tsp xanthan gum
- 1/2 tsp Salt
- Icing
- 1 Cup Cream Cheese 225g / 8 oz
- 3 Tbsp. Powdered Erythritol (So Nourished)
- 1 tsp Vanilla Extract
- 1/2 tsp Lemon Zest

Instructions

1. Separate the egg whites and yolks. Beat the egg whites until they form white peaks.
2. Into the same bowl, place the rest of the cake ingredients (including the egg yolks) into the bowl. Mix until well combined.
3. Pour into a greased loaf tin (9" X 5")
4. Bake at 180 C (355 F) for 45 mins (fan forced)
5. Whilst the cake is in the oven, beat the cream cheese, erythritol, vanilla extract and lemon zest together with an electric beater.
6. Set aside and ice the cake once it has finished cooling.
7. Slice and enjoy

Prep Time: 10 Minutes

Cook Time: 30 Minutes

Servings: 10

Ingredient

- 3/4 Cup Almonds Chopped
- 1 Cup Walnuts Chopped
- 1/2 Cup Sunflower Seeds Chopped
- 1/4 Cup Almond Flakes Chopped
- 1 Tbsp. Chia Seeds
- 1 Tbsp. Flax Seeds
- 1/2 Cup Almond Flour
- 1/2 Cup Desiccated Coconut
- 1 Large Egg
- 1/3 Cup Butter Melted
- 1/4 Cup MCT Oil
- 1/4 Cup Sugar Free Maple Syrup

Instructions

1. Preheat your oven to 180C (360F). Chop all the seeds and nuts into around 4 - 5 pieces each where possible (or pulse 12 times in a food processor). Place into a large bowl.
2. Keto granola in food processor
3. Add the rest of the ingredients into the bowl, and mix around.
4. Keto granola with maple syrup
5. On a baking tray with parchment paper, place the granola out into a flat even layer. Place in the oven for 15 mins.
6. Keto granola on baking sheet
7. Once the timer goes off, pull it out and mix all the ingredients around, making sure that the edges don't burn. Keep putting it in the oven in 5 to 10 min intervals so that the mixture doesn't burn.
8. 30 mins should be enough to make this granola crunchy, but depending on your oven it might be more or less, so please keep an eye on it. It should turn a golden brown all over.

Prep Time: 10 Minutes

Cook Time: 50 Minutes

Servings: 16

Ingredient

- 7 Large Eggs
- 1/2 cup Coconut Flour
- 1/2 cup Butter 120g / 4 oz (use 1/2 cup olive/coconut oil for dairy free)
- 1/4 tsp Salt
- 1/4 tsp baking powder (aluminum free if possible)
- 1/2 tsp xanthan gum (optional)

Instructions

1. Preheat oven to 180 C (355 F).
2. Crack the eggs into a bowl and mix for 1 minute until well combined.
3. Add the coconut flour, butter, salt, baking powder and xanthan gum, and mix until completely combined. The mixture will become quite thick.

4. Line an 8.5 X 5-inch (21.5 x 12.7 cm) loaf tin with parchment paper and pour the batter into the tin. Level the top with a spatula if uneven.

5. Bake for 50 minutes or until a skewer comes out of the middle clean.

6. Nutrition information is for 1 slice. Slice and store in the fridge for up to 5 days or in the freezer for up to 2 weeks. This bread freezes well.

Prep Time: 10 Minutes

Cook Time: 4hrs 2 Minutes

Servings: 12

Ingredient

Base:

- 5 oz Cream Cheese
- 2 oz Butter melted
- 1/4 Cup Refined Coconut Oil 60ml / 2 fl oz melted
- 1 Tbsp. Erythritol (So Nourished)
- 1 tsp Vanilla Extract

Top

- 1/2 Cup Refined Coconut Oil 120ml / 4 fl oz melted
- 2 tsp Erythritol (So Nourished)
- 1 tsp Cocoa Powder

Instructions

1. For the base: In a medium-sized mixing bowl, beat the cream cheese with the butter until combined.

2. Add the coconut oil, erythritol and vanilla, and mix until combined.

3. Divide the mixture between 12 cups of a silicone mini cupcake tray (they should be three-quarters full).

4. Smooth the top with a small teaspoon. Place in the freezer for 20 minutes until relatively hard on top.

5. For the top: In a separate bowl, mix the melted coconut oil with the erythritol and cocoa powder. Pour on top of the semi-frozen base layer, and freeze until completely set, about 4 hours.

Prep Time: 10 Minutes

Cook Time: 10 Minutes

Servings: 12

Ingredient

- 3.5 oz Salted Butter (3.5 oz – 1/2 cup)
- 4.5 oz Erythritol (So Nourished) (4.5 oz – 3/4 cup)
- 1 tsp Vanilla Extract
- 1 large Egg (50g / 1.7 oz)
- 6 oz Almond Flour (6 oz – 170g) by weight, equals about 1 1/2 cups, depending on your almond flour
- 1/2 tsp baking powder
- 1/2 tsp xanthan gum
- 1/4 tsp Salt
- 3 oz Sugar Free Chocolate Chips (90g – 3/4 cup)

Instructions

1. Preheat a fan forced oven to 180C (360F).
2. Melt the butter in saucepan until melted and hot over medium heat. Place the melted butter and erythritol in

a mixing bowl and beat until combined. Add the vanilla and egg, and beat on low for another 15 seconds.

3. Add the almond flour, baking powder, xanthan gum and salt. Beat until well combined.

4. Press the dough together and remove from the bowl. Knead in the chocolate chips with your hands or a silicone spatula.

5. Use a small ice cream scoop to divide and shape the dough into 12 portions and place on a lined baking tray. Bake for 10-12 minutes at 180C (360F). The cookies will look a little undercooked when removing from the oven, but after cooling they will harden.

6. Baking tip if cookies have not flattened after 6-7 minutes in the oven, press down with the back of a fork.

7. Allow to cool for 15 minutes before serving. Keep in an airtight container for up to 7 days.

Prep Time: 15 Minutes

Cook Time: 40 Minutes

Servings: 16

Ingredient

- 7 Large Eggs (50g / 1.7 oz each)
- 3.5 oz Butter melted (100 g / 1/2 cup)
- 1 oz Coconut Oil (30 g / 2 Tbsp.)
- 7 oz Almond Flour (200 g / 2 Cups)
- 1 teaspoon baking powder (5g / 0.2 oz)
- 1/2 teaspoon xanthan gum (2g)
- 1/2 teaspoon Salt (2g)

Instructions

1. Preheat the oven to 180 C (355 F).
2. Put the eggs in a bowl and beat on high for 1 to 2 minutes.
3. Add the melted butter and coconut oil, and beat until smooth.

4. Add the almond flour, baking powder, xanthan gum and salt, and beat until combined and thick.

5. Scrape into an 8-inch X 4-inch (20 cm x 10 cm) loaf pan lined with baking paper.

6. Bake for 45 minutes or until a skewer comes out of the middle clean.

7. Slice into 16 thin slices and store in an airtight container in the fridge for up to 7 days or up to 1 month in the freezer.

Prep Time: 10 Minutes

Cook Time: 10 Minutes

Servings: 12

Ingredient

- 3.5 oz Salted Butter (3.5 oz – 1/2 cup)
- 4.5 oz Erythritol (So Nourished) (4.5 oz – 3/4 cup)
- 1 tsp Vanilla Extract
- 1 large Egg (50g / 1.7 oz)
- 6 oz Almond Flour (6 oz – 170g) by weight, equals about 1 1/2 cups, depending on your almond flour
- 1/2 tsp baking powder
- 1/2 tsp xanthan gum
- 1/4 tsp Salt
- 3 oz Sugar Free Chocolate Chips (90g – 3/4 cup)

Instructions

1. Preheat a fan forced oven to 180C (360F).
2. Melt the butter in saucepan until melted and hot over medium heat. Place the melted butter and erythritol in

a mixing bowl and beat until combined. Add the vanilla and egg, and beat on low for another 15 seconds.

3. Add the almond flour, baking powder, xanthan gum and salt. Beat until well combined.

4. Press the dough together and remove from the bowl. Knead in the chocolate chips with your hands or a silicone spatula.

5. Use a small ice cream scoop to divide and shape the dough into 12 portions and place on a lined baking tray. Bake for 10-12 minutes at 180C (360F). The cookies will look a little undercooked when removing from the oven, but after cooling they will harden.

6. Baking tip if cookies have not flattened after 6-7 minutes in the oven, press down with the back of a fork.

7. Allow to cool for 15 minutes before serving. Keep in an airtight container for up to 7 days.

Prep Time: 20 Minutes

Cook Time: 15 Minutes

Servings: 2

Ingredient

- 2 sweet potatoes unpeeled (about 300g), sliced into 1 inch thick wedges or fries
- 1.5 tbsp olive oil
- 2 salmon fillets 250g
- 1/2 cup petit poi's 65g – or regular peas

Green Dressing:

- 1 garlic clove minced
- 1/2 tbsp capers drained
- 1 small gherkin finely chopped (25g)
- 1/3 tsp Dijon
- 2 tbsp olive oil
- 2 tbsp fresh parsley finely chopped
- 1/2 medium lemon, juiced

Tartar Sauce:

- 1/3 cup Greek yogurt 80g
- 1½ tbsp mini capers drained
- 1/2 tsp lemon juice
- 1 small green onion very finely chopped
- 1 tbsp fresh parsley finely chopped, plus extra to serve
- Salt and pepper to taste

Instructions

1. Preheat the oven to 400F / 200C /180 fan.
2. Put the sweet potatoes in a large roasting tray lined with greaseproof paper. Drizzle with 1 tbsp olive oil and season with salt. Roast for 25 – 35 minutes, turning half way through, or until soft to your liking.
3. Sweet potato chips
4. Place all the green dressing ingredients in amini food processor (or I find spice grinder works fab for this) and blitz until smooth. For a chunkier dressing you can just mix in a bowl.
5. Mix all the ingredients for tartar sauce together in a small bowl.
6. Season the salmon with salt and pepper. Add 1/2 tbsp. of olive oil to a nonstick frying pan and fan fry skin side down for 4 minutes. Flip and cook for a further 4 – 5

minutes, or until the salmon is cooked through. Cooking times will vary depending on the thickness of your salmon.

7. Add peas to a mug of boiling water and allow to thaw for 5 minutes. Option to boil in a little water for 2 – 3 minutes until cooked. Drain.

8. Plate sweet potatoes, salmon and peas and drizzle with dressing. Serve with tartar sauce on the side.

11. Keto Pumpkin Soup

Prep Time: 20 Minutes

Cook Time: 15 Minutes

Servings: 2

Ingredient

- 750 g pumpkin
- 1 small yellow onion diced (70g)
- 3 cloves garlic minced (12g)
- 1 tbsp extra virgin olive oil
- 2.5 tbsp butter ghee or more olive oil
- 1 tsp sea salt or to taste
- 1/3 tsp cracked black pepper or to taste
- 1.1 L chicken stock or veggie stock

Optional To Serve:

- 1 tbsp heavy cream
- 1 tsp chili flakes or to taste
- Pinch of cracked black pepper

Instructions

1. Preheat the oven to 400F / 200°C / 180 fan.
2. Chop the pumpkin in half and remove the seeds. Peel
    (you don't need to if using Hokkaido or delicate) and
    chop into 2cm chunks. Place the pumpkin on a baking
    tray lined with greaseproof paper. Drizzle with 1 tbsp
    olive oil and a pinch of salt. Cook for 35 minutes until
    soft, turning once during cooking.

Pumpkin:

1. Add the butter, ghee or more olive oil to a sauce pan.
    Fry the onions for 3 minutes on a medium heat until
    soft and translucent. Add the garlic for 30 seconds until
    fragrant.
2. Pumpkin soup
3. Add the pumpkin and stock to a saucepan and simmer
    for 20 minutes on a medium/ low heat. Use a blender
    like a Vitamin to blitz until smooth.
4. Soup
5. Adjust the seasoning to taste and serve with an optional
    drizzle of cream, chili flakes and more cracked black
    pepper.

Prep Time: 10 Minutes

Cook Time: 1hr 10 Minutes

Servings: 6

Ingredient

Instant Pot:

- 1 medium chicken 1.4kg (whole)
- 1/2 bulb garlic flavoring only
- 1 small onion flavoring only (70g)
- 15 g parsley flavoring only
- 2 ribs celery flavoring only
- 1 tsp salt
- 1/2 tsp cracked black pepper
- 3 L water

Buffalo sauce:

- 1 bottle Franks hot sauce 148g
- 1/4 cup butter or ghee melted (57g)
- 1/2 tsp garlic powder
- 1 tsp onion powder
- 1/2 tsp salt or to taste

- 1/2 tsp pepper or to taste

To serve:

- 1 – 2 tbsp olive oil
- 2 tbsp chopped fresh parsley
- Mayo on the side

Instructions

Instant Pot Method:

1. Place all the ingredients listed under Instant Pot in the pot.
2. Cook for 1 hour on manual high (making sure the valve is sealed). Once cooked, release the valve and allow to slowly release for 10 minutes or until you can remove the lid.
3. Meanwhile, mix sauce ingredients together in a bowl until combined.
4. Remove the chicken from the Instant Pot using a slotted spoon and place on a chopping board. Pull the chicken apart slightly with a fork to allow it to cool. Cool enough to be able to touch with your hands. Shred using two forks or your hands, discarding any bones, gristle and excess skin (but keep a little bit of the skin

to be crisped up under the broiler – best bit, right guys?)

5. Place the shredded meat on a nonstick baking tray.

6. Drain the juices from the instant pot, discarding the vegetables. I used a gravy strainer here to re-move the fat too.

7. Add 1/4 cup of the stock and 2 tbsp of olive oil to the meat in the tray and toss to combine. Broil for 5 minutes.

8. Add the sauce and toss through the chicken. Broil for a further 8 – 10 minutes, or until the crispiness is to your liking. Turn twice during broiling.

9. To serve, top with fresh parsley or coriander, an optional drizzle of olive oil and mayo.

10. Add the remaining stock to a saucepan and simmer for about 10 – 15 minutes until con-cent rated. Store or use as a gravy.

Oven Method

1. Preheat the oven to 400F / 200C / 180 fan. Place the chicken on a trivet in a roasting tin, removing the string. Season the chicken, stuff with parsley and rub with 1 tbsp of olive oil. Add the onion, gar lic and celery with 1 cup of water to the tray.

2. Cover the chicken with foil for 1 hour.

3. Remove the foil and continue cooking for a further 20 – 30 minutes, or cook to the package instructions depending on the size of your bird, until the skin is golden, and the juices run clear when you insert a skewer. Depending on the size of your chicken you may need to adjust the timings. On average, 25 minutes per 500g plus 25 minutes to crisp up the skin.

4. Place the chicken on a chopping board. Pull the chicken slightly apart to cool and allow to rest for 10 minutes and then shred the meat using 2 forks / your hands. Discard any bones, gristle etc. and place the meat on a non-stick baking tray.

5. Drain the juices from the tray discarding the vegetables. I used a gravy strainer here to remove the fat too.

6. Add 1/4 cup of the stock and 2 tbsp of olive oil to the meat in the tray and toss to combine. Broil for 5 minutes.

7. Add the sauce and toss through the chicken. Broil for a further 8 – 10 minutes, or until is crisped to your liking. Turn twice during broiling.

8. To serve, top with fresh parsley or coriander and an optional drizzle of olive oil and mayo.

Prep Time: 10 Minutes

Cook Time: 30 Minutes

Servings: 6

Ingredient

- 800 g Chicken Thigh skin removed, approximately 6 medium size
- 180 g Prosciutto thinly sliced
- 1 cup Thickened Cream (heavy whipping cream)
- 1/4 cup chicken stock or bone broth
- 2 cloves garlic crushed
- 1 tsp black pepper

Instructions

1. Preheat your oven to 180C (350F)
2. Bring a frying pan to a medium high heat, and place the chicken thighs top side down to cook until golden brown in color (5-10 minutes). Turn and cook until the internal temperature of the chicken is 73C (165F)

Cooked chicken thigh:

1. Remove the chicken from the frying pan, wrap in prosciutto and add back to the pan, cooking on all sides for a further 2-3 minutes or until crispy. Remove from the pan.
2. Cooked chicken thigh wrapped
3. Reduce to a low heat, and add cream, stock, pepper and garlic. Stir to incorporate the remaining chicken fat into the sauce, then place the chicken thigh back into the sauce.

Before oven:

1. Place into the oven for 5-10 minutes, or until the sauce has reduced to your liking.
2. Cooked sauce
3. Will keep in the fridge for up to 4 days, or can be frozen for up to 2 months.

Prep Time: 10 Minutes

Cook Time: 20 Minutes

Servings: 4

Ingredient

- 1 Tbsp fennel seeds
- ½ tsp salt
- 5 cloves garlic divided
- ¼ cup butter 2 oz/70 g (or olive oil for dairy free)
- 4 pork chops 2 lb/800 g approx.
- ½ lb green beans 250 g, trimmed
- 1 lemon sliced
- 2 Tbsp olive oil
- Salt and ground black pepper

Instructions

1. Line a 15-inch X 10-inch (38 cm X 25 cm) baking sheet with a piece of parchment paper. Preheat a broiler (grill) to 200 C (180 fan forced).

2. In a mortar and pestle, grind the fennel seeds and salt together until a rough powder forms. Add in 2 cloves of the garlic and finely crush them. Melt the butter and place in a bowl. Stir in the fennel and garlic mixture.

3. Place the pork chops on the baking sheet and rub the tops with the infused butter.

4. Place the green beans, remaining garlic, and lemon slices beside the chops. Drizzle with the olive oil and season with salt and pepper to taste.

5. Roast for 20 minutes or until the internal temperature of the pork reaches 74 C (165 F).

6. Remove from the oven and allow to rest for 5 minutes before serving.

7. Oven roasted pork chops

Prep Time: 5 Minutes

Cook Time: 45 Minutes

Servings: 6

Ingredient

- 12 slices streaky bacon chopped (200g)
- 2 tbsp olive oil
- 1 tbsp butter
- 2 cloves garlic
- 1 small yellow onion 70g
- 2/3 cup heavy cream
- 1/2 cup cream cheese 120g
- 1/2 cup grated mozzarella 56g (or cheddar)
- 1/2 cup grated parmesan 30g
- 2 tbsp water to thin
- 1.5 tsp dijon mustard
- 1/4 tsp black pepper cracked or to taste
- Salt to taste
- 1 large cauliflower 470g (or 6 baby cauliflowers)
- Option to top with fresh thyme

Instructions

1. Preheat oven 392F / 200C / 180 fan.
2. Add the bacon to non-stick frying pan and cook for 3 minutes. Add the butter and olive oil, onion, garlic, sea salt and black pepper and sauté for 3 more minutes until the onions are soft. Remove from the pan and set side.
3. Add the heavy cream, cream cheese, mozzarella,1/4 cup Parmesan cheese, mustard, 2 tbsp water and seasoning into the pan. Mix until combined using a spatula or hand balloon whisk. Reduce the heat to medium/ low and simmer until the sauce thickens. Once thick, stir in the bacon and onion. Taste and adjust the seasoning to taste.
4. Slice the cauliflower into 1/2 cm thick slices. I used a mandolin to get them nice and even and baby cauliflowers but you can use a larger one and just break into large florets and slice. You can use the ends too so as not to waste them.
5. Grease an oven proof cast iron pan or gratin dish with a little butte (mine was 10 inch x 2 inches). Add a thin layer of sauce on the bottom, followed by some cauliflower slices, more sauce, another layer of cauliflower and top with a final layer of sauce and

sprinkle the remaining parmesan over the top of the dish. Depending on the size of your dish you may prefer to have 1 or 2 layers of cauliflower and 2 or 3 layers of sauce.

6. Cover with foil and bake for 20 minutes. Uncover and cook for a further 15 minutes or until golden on top and the cauliflower is tender. Option to top with fresh thyme for prettiness.

Prep Time: 5 Minutes

Cook Time: 20 Minutes

Servings: 2

Ingredient

- 200 g cherry tomatoes or perino tomatoes
- 100 g feta cheese or white danish style cheese
- 1 Tbsp olive oil
- 1/2 tsp salt and pepper
- 1 tsp dried chili or harissa spice mix
- 3 cloves garlic reduce if you like a mild garlic flavor
- 1 packet keto alternative noodles slender or konjack noodles
- grated parmesan cheese to serve

Instructions

1. Preheat your fan-forced oven to 200C (400F) (220C or 420F if non fan forced)
2. Into a medium baking tray, place the tomatoes, and cover with 1/2 the olive oil. Mix until well combined.

3. Tomatoes covered with olive oil

4. Add the salt, pepper, and dried chili (I used harrissa spice mix which is also fantastic). Mix until well coated.

5. Make a gap between the tomatoes, and place the feta cheese into the middle. Place the remaining olive oil over the cheese along with the garlic, and place into the oven for 20 minutes.

6. Cook 4 servings of the pasta of your choice according to the direction. If using the black bean fettuccini, boil a pot of water and cook for 7 minutes or until your desired texture. Drain and set aside.

7. Remove the baked feta and tomato dish from the oven, and using two forks press mixture together until it's all well combined.

8. Place the cooked pasta into the baked feta dish, and mix until the pasta is well coated in the cheese tomato sauce. Serve with a sprinkle of parmesan cheese

9. Keto baked feta pasta

Prep Time: 15 Minutes

Cook Time: 30 Minutes

Servings: 10

Ingredient

- 350 ml egg whites or egg whites from 12 large eggs – 12 floz
- 60 g whey protein powder 2 scoops, unflavored – 2 oz
- 1/2 tsp Cream of Tartar
- butter for greasing the pan

Instructions

1. Preheat your convection (fan forced) oven to 160C (320F).
2. In a large clean dry bowl, whisk the egg whites on medium speed until stiff peaks form (about 5-8 minutes). This can be done in a stand mixer or using a hand held electric mixer.

3. Add in the whey protein powder and Cream of Tartar, and mix on low until all the ingredients are combined and uniform in color.

4. Grease a bread loaf tin, and line with parchment paper (quick tip, scrunching the parchment paper into a ball, then unfolding will help the paper mould to the shape of the tin).

5. Spoon the egg white mixture into the bread loaf tin until the mixture goes above the top of the tin. Use the back of your spoon to shape into a bread loaf, and bake in the oven for 30 minutes

6. Once 30 minutes is up, turn the oven off and place a kitchen towel into the door of the oven to keep it slightly adjar. Keep it like this for 20-30 minutes, as this will allow the oven to cool slowly and help avoid the loaf from deflating.

7. Remove the loaf from the oven, and slice into 10 thick slices. Nutritional information is per slice.

8. These slices will keep in the fridge for up to 3 days, or frozen with parchment paper between the slices for up to 2 weeks.

Prep Time: 10 Minutes

Cook Time: 1hr 3 Minutes

Servings: 8

Ingredient

- 3 batches of 90 second keto bread
- 1 large onion peeled + quartered (80g)
- 3 Tbsp butter or olive oil (DF)
- 450 g Italian or Toulouse sausages roughly 3 large or ground pork mince (f using pork meat add 2 extra cloves of garlic + 1/2 tsp extra of each herb)
- 3 rashers smoked streaky bacon diced small (60g)
- 1 whole lemon zest
- 1/2 tsp flaked sea salt
- 1/2 tsp coarse black pepper
- 2 sticks celery diced small (80g)
- 2/3 cup cauliflower florets diced small (90g)
- 1 clover garlic minced
- 2 tbsp fresh sage finely chopped
- 1 tbsp fresh rosemary finely chopped
- 1 tbsp fresh thyme leaves

- 2/3 – 3/4 cup chicken stock
- 1 large egg

Instructions

1. Preheat the oven to 320F / 160C / 140 fan.
2. Make the keto bread as per my recipe. Place on a greaseproof line baking tray and partially dry out for about 10 – 15 minutes. Remove from the oven and allow to cool whilst you make the meat filling.
3. Blitz the onions in a food processor until finely chopped, or chop fine with a knife then tip into a large bowl.
4. If using sausages, remove skins and break up the meat.
5. Place sausages into the food processor (with the onions) and add the bacon, seasoning and lemon zest.
6. Pulse until combined.
7. Add 1 tbsp of butter or olive oil to a non-stick frying pan and fry the sausage mix until cooked through, about 8 minutes. Set aside.
8. Add 2 butter or olive oil to the same pan. Add the celery, cauliflower, garlic and herbs and cook for 4 – 5 minutes until the cauliflower is soft. Option to add some water if the mix starts to get dry.

9. Remove from the heat. Add cooked sausage meat to the cauliflower mix and stir to combine.

10. Mix the egg and stock in a small bowl. Add croutons and egg mix to the sausage mix and toss well to combine making sure the croutons are covered.

11. Turn up the oven to 374F / 190C / 170 fan.

12. Grease a baking tin with oil or butter. Add the stuffing mix and bake for about 45 minutes (giving it a good stir about half way through) or until the sausage meat is set and the croutons are golden. Start checking it from about 30 minutes.

13. Garnish with a good drizzle of olive oil and fresh parsley.

Prep Time: 00 Minutes

Cook Time: 00 Minutes

Servings: 8

Ingredient

- 1 tsp salt and pepper or to taste

- 1.8 kg boneless turkey breast

- 4 tbsp butter or olive oil

- 3 garlic cloves minced

- 1.5 tbsp finely chopped fresh rosemary

- 1 tbsp thyme leaves + 3 sprigs to serve

- 1/2 lemon + zest

- 1 medium onion quartered (100g)

- 2 bay leaves optional

- 3/4 cup white wine

- 7.1 oz cubed bacon lardoons pancetta or streaky bacon, sliced / 200g

- 14 oz Brussels sprouts halved / 400g

- 1 large head broccoli cut into small florets 10oz / 290g

- 2 tbsp fresh parsley chopped

Instructions

1. Rub the turkey in 1 tsp of salt the day before and place
    in the fridge covered with tin foil.
2. Combine lemon zest, rosemary, thyme and garlic with
    melted butter or olive oil in a small bowl and mix to
    combine.
3. Using your hands work your way between the breast
    meat and the skin, lifting it up and pushing 1/3 of the
    mix in-between. Rub the rest all over the joint. Season
    with black pepper all over.
4. Put the onion in the base of a large roasting tin with the
    optional bay leaves. Sit the turkey breast on top with
    the half lemon in the tin. Cover with a loose tent of tin
    foil (if making the day before place in the fridge). Take
    the turkey out of the fridge 1 hour before roasting.
5. Preheat the oven to 374F / 190C / 170 fan. Cooking
    times vary depending on the weight of your turkey and
    how hot your oven runs. Based on 25 – 30 minutes per
    500g. Mine was a 1.8kg breast and took about 1.5
    hours. The veggies + bacon will take 30 – 40 minutes.
6. Put the turkey covered in foil in the oven for 1 hour.
    Remove the foil and baste in juices. Remove most of the
    juices leaving just a little in the pan (use this as a base
    for your gravy).

7. Add the wine to the tin around the turkey, along with the sprouts, broccoli and bacon, toss well and return to the oven UNCOVERED for 30 – 40 minutes (alter timings based on weight of turkey knowing the veggies take 30 – 40 minutes depending on how crisp you like them). Give them a stir half way through cooking.

8. Take the pan out of the oven. Option to add a little of the reserved stock to the veggies too and cover to keep warm. Transfer the turkey to a board and rest covered with foil for 15 – 20 minutes before slicing. Use the juices to make any gravy.

9. For super crispy take the skin off the joint before carving it. Spread on baking tray and return to oven 400F / 200C 10 – 20 minutes turning once. You can also remove the fatty underside of the skin to crisp up even more. Be warned though the skin will shrink so if you then place it back on top it will be a little smaller… but so totally worth it for that epic skin in my book! Just Slice it up and serve on the side with the meat.

10. Carve the turkey (put the veggies back in the oven for a couple of minutes to warm through if gone cold).

11. Garnish the turkey and veggies with fresh parsley and thyme. Option to squeeze over the roasted lemon and serve with keto stuffing and your own gravy.

Prep Time: 10 Minutes

Cook Time: 35 Minutes

Servings: 4

Ingredient

- 4 medium sweet potatoes 840g
- 2 large chicken breasts or 320g roasted chicken
- 1 tsp extra virgin olive oil
- 1 large avocado
- 1 large lime juiced
- Salt and pepper to taste
- 2 green onions finely sliced (30g)
- 2 – 3 tbsp fresh cilantro chopped (10g)
- 1 medium green jalapeño chopped

Instructions

1. Avocado mix.
2. Slice sweet potatoes, option to fluff the insides a little with a fork and add a drizzle of olive oil Preheat the

oven to 425F / 220C / 180 fan and line a large baking sheet with parchment paper.

3. Scrub your sweet potatoes and dry with kitchen roll. Rub the skins with a little olive oil and optional salt. Prick with a fork several times to release any steam.

4. Add sweet potatoes to the baking sheet and bake for 45 – 55 minutes or until soft. Cooking times will vary depending on the size of your potatoes. (To speed up the cooking time you can precook in the microwave for 6 – 8 minutes then cook for about 20 minutes in the oven if you prefer.)

5. Meanwhile, if you're cooking the chicken, drizzle with oil and sprinkle with sea salt, then bake on a separate parchment lined baking sheet for about 20 minutes, or until no longer pink on the inside. Allow to rest and then shred the meat using 2 forks. Option to use chicken thighs if you prefer.

6. Chicken on a baking tray

7. Mix the avocado with lime juice, salt, pepper, green onions, cilantro and jalapeño. Adjust jalapeño quantity, lime juice and seasoning to taste.

8. Avocado in a bowl

9. Mix chicken with if you like then top with chicken mix and more cilantro.

Prep Time: 10 Minutes

Cook Time: 10 Minutes

Servings: 2

Ingredient

- Slaw Dressing
- 1/4 cup unsweetened Greek or coconut yoghurt for dairy free
- 1/2 tsp extra virgin olive oil
- 1/2 tsp lemon juice
- Pinch of salt + pepper

Slaw:

- 1/2 cup red cabbage shredded (35g)
- 1 cup white cabbage shredded (70g)
- 1 small carrot peeled + shredded (50g)
- 1 scallion finely sliced (15g)
- 20 g mange tout thinly sliced
- 2 tbsp fresh parsley finely chopped

Salmon:

- 1 tbsp extra virgin olive oil
- 1/2 tsp paprika
- 1/3 tsp garlic powder or 2 garlic cloves minced
- 1/4 tsp salt
- 1/4 tsp black pepper
- 2 5-ounce salmon fillets

Instructions

1. Mix the slaw dressing together in a small bowl. Season to taste.
2. Add all the slaw vegetable ingredients to a mixing bowl and toss to combine with the dressing. Place in the fridge whilst you make the salmon.
3. Cabbage slaw in white bowl
4. Add 1 tbsp olive oil, paprika, garlic powder, salt and pepper to a small bowl. Stir to combine.
5. Rinse the salmon fillets and pat dry thoroughly with paper towels. Brush marinade on top of salmon.
6. Salmon
7. Spray a non-stick frying pan with a little olive oil. Cook flesh side down (skin side up) undisturbed for 3 – 4 minutes on a medium heat. Flip and cook for a further

5 minutes or until the salmon is cooked through to your liking. NOTE: Cooking times will vary depending on the thickness of your fillets and if you use wild or farmed salmon.

8. Salmon in pan

9. Option to bake in the oven on a greaseproof lined baking tray for 12 – 15 minutes. (375F / 190C) NOTE: oven roasting often results in the albumin releasing from the salmon (white substance you often see on salmon). This is perfectly safe to eat. Even cooking at low temperatures I find it does it so if you want pretty salmon my advice is to pan fry!

10. Serve salmon with slaw. Sprinkle the fresh parsley and lemon wedges.

11. Salmon slaw

Prep Time: 20 Minutes

Cook Time: 15 Minutes

Servings: 2

Ingredient

- 2 sweet potatoes unpeeled (about 300g), sliced into 1 inch thick wedges or fries
- 1.5 tbsp olive oil
- 2 salmon fillets 250g
- 1/2 cup petit pois 65g – or regular peas

Green Dressing:

- 1 garlic clove minced
- 1/2 tbsp capers drained
- 1 small gherkin finely chopped (25g)
- 1/3 tsp Dijon
- 2 tbsp olive oil
- 2 tbsp fresh parsley finely chopped
- 1/2 medium lemon, juiced

Tartar Sauce:

- 1/3 cup Greek yogurt 80g
- 1½ tbsp mini capers drained
- 1/2 tsp lemon juice
- 1 small green onion very finely chopped
- 1 tbsp fresh parsley finely chopped, plus extra to serve
- Salt and pepper to taste

Instructions

1. Preheat the oven to 400F / 200C /180 fan.
2. Put the sweet potatoes in a large roasting tray lined with greaseproof paper. Drizzle with 1 tbsp olive oil and season with salt. Roast for 25 − 35 minutes, turning half way through, or until soft to your liking.
3. Sweet potato chips
4. Place all the green dressing ingredients in amini food processor (or I find spice grinder works fab for this) and blitz until smooth. For a chunkier dressing you can just mix in a bowl.
5. Mix all the ingredients for tartar sauce together in a small bowl.
6. Season the salmon with salt and pepper. Add 1/2 tbsp of olive oil to a non-stick frying pan and fan fry skin side down for 4 minutes. Flip and cook for a further 4

– 5 minutes, or until the salmon is cooked through. Cooking times will vary depending on the thickness of your salmon.

7. Add peas to a mug of boiling water and allow to thaw for 5 minutes. Option to boil in a little water for 2 – 3 minutes until cooked. Drain.

8. Plate sweet potatoes, salmon and peas and drizzle with dressing. Serve with tartar sauce on the side.

Prep Time: 5 Minutes

Cook Time: 15 Minutes

Servings: 3

Ingredient

- 500 g Beef Mince (Ground Beef) (1 lb)
- 1/2 Whole Brown Onion
- 1 Tbsp Gluten Free Soy Sauce
- 2 Tbsp Sesame Oil
- 1 tsp ground ginger
- 2 tsp Fish Sauce
- 1 tsp Siracha Sauce
- 300 g Dry Slaw (Cabbage Mix)
- 5 Tbsp Homemade Mayonnaise
- 2 tsp Dijon Mustard

Instructions

1. Heat a frying pan up to a medium / high heat

2. Dice the onion and add both the onion and the beef mince to the pan. Cook until the mince goes slightly brown and the onion becomes soft.

3. Add the soy sauce, ginger, sesame seed oil, and siracha and fish sauce to the mince. Let it simmer for 2 mins

4. Add the dry slaw mix to the frying pan and let it simmer whilst the cabbage begins to break down and become soft.

5. Mix the mayonnaise and the Dijon mustard together, and add to the frying pan, mix around quickly and serve.

Prep Time: 5 Minutes

Cook Time: 15 Minutes

Servings: 4

Ingredient

- 500 g Ground Beef 1.2 lb
- 300 g Package Dry Coleslaw (green & red cabbage) (10oz)
- 2 cloves garlic minced
- 3 Tbsp Sesame Seed Oil
- 1 Tbsp Fish Sauce
- 2 Tbsp soy sauce or coconut amino
- 4 Tbsp Sesame Seeds topping
- Salt and pepper to taste

Instructions

1. Heat sesame seed oil in a frying pan (or wok)
2. Add in ground beef (beef mince) and cook for 10 mins.
3. Add the remaining ingredients, with a pinch of salt and pepper. Cook for another 5 mins.

4. Serve into 4 meal prep containers. Store in the refrigerator for up to 4 days.

Prep Time: 20 Minutes

Cook Time: 15 Minutes

Servings: 5

Ingredient

- 500 g Chicken Thighs 1.2 lb
- 2 tsp Salt
- 2 tsp ground paprika and more for garnish
- 2 tbsp olive oil
- 2 medium Bell Peppers Capsicum
- 1/2 medium Cauliflower or 4 servings of riced cauliflower
- 2 tsp Tabasco Sauce (optional)
- 2 medium Avocados
- Salt and Pepper to taste

Instructions

1. Place the chicken thighs on a plate and season each side with the salt and paprika.

2. Heat a frying pan set over medium-high heat and add the olive oil. Cook each piece of chicken for 5 minutes on each side, or until cooked through. Remove the chicken from the pan and slice into strips.

3. Return the pan to medium-high heat. Dice the bell peppers and cook for 5 minutes in remaining pan oils.

4. Chop the cauliflower into florets and then into rice-sized pieces. Alternatively, you can purchase cauliflower rice or pulse the florets in a food processor.

5. Divide the cauliflower rice between meal prep containers. Top with the Tabasco sauce (if using) and paprika. Top with the cooked chicken and bell peppers.

6. Halve and pit the avocados, and scoop the flesh into a small bowl. Mash the avocado and season with paprika, Tabasco sauce (if using), salt and pepper. Dollop onto each portion or keep separately.

7. Store in the fridge for up to 4 days.

Prep Time: 10 Minutes

Cook Time: 20 Minutes

Servings: 4

Ingredient

- 1 Litre Chicken Stock
- 1/2 Large Broccoli Bunch chopped
- 1/2 Onion diced
- 1 Cloves garlic crushed
- 1 Cup heavy whipping cream
- 1/3 Cup grated parmesan cheese
- 1 Cup Aged Cheddar
- 2 Tbsp olive oil
- 4 Slices Prosciutto
- Salt to taste

Instructions

1. In a large pot, add the olive oil, chopped onion, and garlic. Cook on medium heat until the onion is translucent.

2. Add the chopped broccoli and the chicken stock to the pot, and cook for 10 mins until the broccoli becomes tender

3. Using an immersion blender, remove the pot from the heat, and blend in the pot until smooth.

4. Place back on heat, adding the cheese, cream and salt.

5. In a frying pan, heat to medium and cook the prosciutto for 2 mins eat side until slightly crispy. Be careful not to burn.

6. Serve in bowls, topped with extra cream, a few pine nuts and the crispy prosciutto.

Prep Time: 15 Minutes

Cook Time: 30 Minutes

Servings: 4

Ingredient

- 500 g Organic Tofu (1 lb)
- 1/3 cup Coconut Oil
- 1 tsp Ginger grated
- 1 medium Onion thinly sliced
- 2 Tbsp soy sauce
- 1 Tbsp Erythritol
- 1 tsp Sesame Oil
- 1/2 cup water
- 1 shallot chopped
- 1 tsp Toasted sesame seeds garnish
- 1/2 Medium Cauliflower (riced)

Instructions

1. Slice the cauliflower into small pieces (rice-sized pieces) and place in the steamer basket above water. Cook for 10-15 mins.
2. Cut the tofu into large cubes, and pat dry with a paper towel.
3. Place the coconut oil into a frying pan, and fry the tofu, turning onto each side until crispy.
4. Remove the tofu from the pan and add the onion and grated ginger. Cook until transparent.
5. Then, add the soy sauce, erythritol, sesame seed oil, water and the pre-cooked tofu.
6. Let it simmer for 5 mins on low.
7. Serve with cauliflower rice.

Prep Time: 10 Minutes

Cook Time: 20 Minutes

Servings: 1

Ingredient

Base:

- 1/2 Cup Grated Mozzarella
- 1/2 Tbsp Almond Flour
- 1/2 Tbsp Cream Cheese
- 1 Medium Egg
- 1/2 tsp Salt
- 1/2 tsp Pepper

Toppings:

- 1 Tbsp Grated Mozzarella
- 1 Tbsp Passata Sauce Tomato Puree
- 1 tsp Dried Oregano

Instructions

1. Preheat the oven to 390 F (200 C)

2. Put the base mozzarella cheese into a microwave safe bowl and microwave for 90 secs.

3. Mix in the rest of the base ingredients with a fork. Roll out with a rolling pin between 2 sheets of baking paper

4. Put the base in the oven for 7 mins, flip the base and cook the other side for 3 mins

5. Take the pizza out of the oven. Using a tablespoon, smother the pizza base with the tomato sauce.

6. Cover in cheese and oregano and place in the oven for another 7 mins.

Prep Time: 10 Minutes

Cook Time: 10 Minutes

Servings: 2

Ingredient

Broth:

- 500 ml Chicken Stock 17 floz
- 2 Garlic Cloves
- 2 tablespoons Liquid Aminos soy sauce
- 1 tablespoon Worcestershire sauce
- 1 teaspoon Ginger
- ½ teaspoon five spice
- ½ teaspoon chili powder
- 1 teaspoon Erythritol
- 2 tablespoons Sesame Seed Oil

Toppings:

- 2 boiled eggs
- 1 packet miracle noodles
- 4 Pieces Sliced Pork

Optional Pork Ingredients:

- 1/4 Cup Liquid Aminos
- 2 Tablespoons Rice Wine Vinegar
- 3 Garlic Cloves
- 300 g Pork Belly 10.5 oz
- 1 Cup water
- 2 teaspoons Erythritol
- 2 wooden skewers

Instructions

1. In a large saucepan, combine the broth ingredients, and simmer for 10 mins.
2. Pour into 2 bowls and serve warm.
3. If using miracle noodles
4. Dry fry them for 8 minutes before adding to the bowl.
5. If using boiled eggs
6. Heat a pot of water to boiling point, add the eggs and set a timer for 5 minutes.
7. Remove from the water and place into an ice bath for 2 minutes before peeling and halving.
8. If using pork:
9. Preheat your oven to 180C (355F)

10. Combine all ingredients into a small Dutch oven, and roll the pork belly into a circle, poking wooden skewers through the meat to keep it rolled

11. Cook for 40 minutes, remove from the broth and slice into round cuts as shown in the photo.

Prep Time: 10 Minutes

Cook Time: 20 Minutes

Servings: 6

Ingredient

Meatballs:

- 500 g ground pork 1 lb
- 2 Tbsp parmesan cheese
- 1/4 Cup Heavy Whipping Cream Pure Cream
- 1 Large Egg
- 1 Tablespoon Garlic Powder
- 1/2 teaspoon salt
- 1/2 teaspoon pepper
- 1 tsp dried oregano
- 1 Tablespoon Worchester sauce

Garlic Yogurt:

- 1 Cup Greek Yogurt
- 1 Cloves Garlic crushed
- 1/2 tsp Salt
- 1/4 tsp Dried Dill (optional)

Instructions

1. Preheat your oven to 180C (355F)
2. In a large mixing bowl, add all the meatball ingredients and mix around with clean hands.
3. Place baking paper into a large baking tray.
4. Using a tablespoon measure, scoop out a portion, and roll into balls
5. Bake for 10 mins, flip them over and bake for another 10-15 mins until cooked all the way through
6. In a bowl, mix together the yogurt, crushed garlic, salt and dill. Serve with the meatballs and enjoy.

www.ingramcontent.com/pod-product-compliance
Lightning Source LLC
Chambersburg PA
CBHW050051260726
48658CB00005B/1891